Praise for
The Glucose Revolution and The Glucose Revolution Pocket Guides

■

"The concept of the glycemic index has been distorted and bastardized by popular writers and diet gurus. Here, at last, is a book that explains what we know about the glycemic index and its importance in designing a diet for optimum health. Carbohydrates are not all bad. Read the good news about pasta and even—believe it or not—sugar!"
—ANDREW WEIL, M.D., University of Arizona College of Medicine, author of *Spontaneous Healing* and *8 Weeks to Optimum Health*

■

"Forget *Sugar Busters*. Forget *The Zone*. If you want the real scoop on how carbohydrates and sugar affect your body, read this book by the world's leading researchers on the subject. It's the authoritative, last word on choosing foods to control your blood sugar."
—JEAN CARPER, best-selling author of *Miracle Cures, Stop Aging Now!* and *Food—Your Miracle Medicine*

■

"*The Glucose Revolution* is nutrition science for the 21st century. Clearly written, it gives the scientific rationale for why all carbohydrates are not created equal. It is a practical guide for both professionals and patients. The food suggestions and recipes are exciting and tasty."

—RICHARD N. PODELL, M.D., M.P.H., Clinical Professor, Department of Family Medicine, UMDNJ–Robert Wood Johnson Medical School, and co-author of *The G-Index Diet: The Missing Link That Makes Permanent Weight Loss Possible*

■

"Here is at last a book explaining the importance of taking into consideration the glycemic index of foods for overall health, athletic performance, and in reducing the risk of heart disease and diabetes. The book clearly explains that there are different kinds of carbohydrates that work in different ways and why a universal recommendation to 'increase the carbohydrate content of your diet' is plainly simple and scientifically inaccurate. Everyone should put the glycemic index approach into practice."

—ARTEMIS P. SIMOPOULOS, M.D., senior author of *The Omega Diet* and *The Healing Diet* and President, The Center for Genetics, Nutrition and Health, Washington, D.C.

■

"Although the jury is still out on the utility of the glycemic index, many of the curious will benefit from a careful reading of this book, and some will find that the glycemic index is particularly helpful for them. Everyone can enjoy the recipes, some of which are to die for!"

—JOHANNA DWYER, D. Sc., R.D., editor, *Nutrition Today*

OTHER *GLUCOSE REVOLUTION* TITLES

The Glucose Revolution: The Authoritative Guide to the Glycemic Index—The Groundbreaking Medical Discovery

The Glucose Revolution Pocket Guide to Diabetes

The Glucose Revolution Pocket Guide to Losing Weight

The Glucose Revolution Pocket Guide to Sports Nutrition

■

FORTHCOMING:

The Glucose Revolution Pocket Guide to Sugar and Energy

The Glucose Revolution Pocket Guide to Your Heart

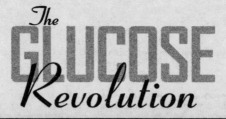

The GLUCOSE Revolution

POCKET GUIDE TO

THE TOP 100
LOW GLYCEMIC FOODS

KAYE FOSTER-POWELL, M. NUTR. & DIET.
JENNIE BRAND-MILLER, PH.D.
THOMAS M.S. WOLEVER, M.D., PH.D.

ADAPTED BY
JOHANNA BURANI, M.S., R.D., C.D.E.
AND LINDA RAO, M.ED.

■

MARLOWE & COMPANY
NEW YORK

Published by
Marlowe & Company
An Imprint of Avalon Publishing Group Incorporated
161 William Street, 16th Floor
New York, NY 10038

The information in this book is intended to help readers make informed decisions about their health and the health of their loved ones. It is not intended to be a substitute for treatment by or the advice and care of a professional health care provider. While the authors and publisher have endeavored to ensure that the information is accurate and up to date, they are not responsible for adverse effects or consequences sustained by any person using this book.

Copyright © text 1998, 2000 Kaye Foster-Powell, Jennie Brand-Miller, Thomas M. S. Wolever.

First published in Australia in 1998 in somewhat different form under the title *Pocket Guide to the G.I. Factor Top 100 Low G.I. Foods* by Hodder Headline Australia Pty Limited.

This edition is published by arrangement with Hodder Headline Australia Pty Limited.

Library of Congress Cataloging-in-Publication Data
Brand-Miller, Janette, 1952-
    [Pocket guide to the top 100 low G.I. foods]
    The glucose revolution pocket guide to the top 100 low glycemic foods / by Jennie Brand-Miller and Kaye Foster-Powell.
    p. cm.
    Published in Australia in 1998 under the title: Pocket guide to the top 100 low G.I. foods.
    ISBN 1-56924-678-5
    1. Glycemic index—Handbooks, manuals, etc. I. Foster-Powell, Kaye. II. Title.

QP701.B73 2000
613.2'83—dc21

99-042190

9 8 7 6
Designed by Pauline Neuwirth, Neuwirth & Associates, Inc.
Distributed by Publishers Group West
Manufactured in the United States of America

CONTENTS

PREFACE

*T*he Glucose Revolution is the definitive, all-in-one guide to the glycemic index (G.I.). Now we have written this pocket guide to answer one of the questions we are asked most frequently: "What foods have the lowest glycemic index values?"

The Glucose Revolution Pocket Guide to the Top 100 Low Glycemic Foods makes it easier than ever to identify those foods that have the lowest G.I. values—and to enjoy them every day, at every meal—for better blood sugar control, weight loss, heart health, peak athletic performance, and overall well-being.

This book offers more in-depth information about the top 100 low G.I. foods than we had room to include in *The Glucose Revolution*. But this book has been written to be read alongside *The Glucose Revolution,* so in the event you haven't already consulted that book, please be sure to do so, for a more comprehensive discussion of the glycemic index and all its uses.

Chapter 1

WHAT THE GLYCEMIC INDEX IS ALL ABOUT

HOW YOU CAN BENEFIT FROM
LOW G.I. FOODS

INCLUDING LOW G.I. FOODS
IN YOUR MEALS

LOW G.I. SUBSTITUTES

STARCH AND THE GLYCEMIC INDEX

MEASURING THE GLYCEMIC INDEX

*W*hat if we were to tell you that eating more of certain foods—certain *delicious* foods— would help you lose weight, manage your diabetes and help protect against heart disease? Sound too good to be true? It's not! The foods we're talking about are specific types of carbohydrates. What's so special about these carbohydrates, you ask? Read on.

Worldwide research since the early 1980s has shown us that different carbohydrate foods have dramatically different effects on blood sugar levels. Until very recently, food scientists and nutritionists widely believed that complex carbohydrates, such as rice and potato, were slowly digested energy foods that caused only a small rise in our blood sugar levels.

Scientists viewed sugars, on the other hand, as villians that cause rapid fluctuations in blood sugar levels. Our glycemic index research has turned all these beliefs upside down and changed the way we think about carbohydrates—forever.

When scientists began to study the actual blood sugar responses to different foods in hundreds of people, they found that many starchy foods (such as bread and potatoes) are digested and absorbed very quickly and that many sugar-containing foods were actually quite slowly absorbed. That was quite a surprise!

THE PANCREAS PRODUCES INSULIN

The pancreas is a vital organ near the stomach, and its main job is to produce the hormone insulin. Carbohydrate stimulates the secretion of insulin more than any other component of food. The slow absorption of the carbohydrate in our food means that the pancreas doesn't have to work so hard and needs to produce less insulin. If the pancreas is overstimulated over a long period of time, it may become "exhausted" and type 2 diabetes can develop in genetically susceptible people. Even without diabetes, high insulin levels are undesirable because they increase the risk of heart disease.

Unfortunately, over time, we have begun to eat more "refined" foods and fewer "whole" foods. This new way of eating has brought with it higher blood sugar levels after a meal and higher insulin responses, as well. Though our bodies do need insulin for carbohydrate metabolism, high levels of the hormone have a profound effect on the development of many diseases. In fact, medical experts now believe that high insulin levels are one of the key factors responsible for heart disease and hypertension. Insulin influences the way we metabolize foods, determining whether we burn fat or carbohydrate to meet our energy needs and ultimately determining whether we store fat in our bodies.

The glycemic index (or G.I.) was developed to rank foods based on their immediate effect on our blood sugar levels. Carbohydrate foods that break down quickly during digestion have the highest G.I. values because the blood sugar response is fast and high. In other words the glucose (or sugar) in the bloodstream increases rapidly. Conversely, carbohydrates that break down slowly, releasing glucose gradually into the bloodstream, have low G.I. values. The substance that produces the greatest rise in blood sugar levels is pure glucose itself. All other foods have less effect when fed in equal amounts of carbohydrate. The glycemic index of pure glucose is set at 100 and every other food is ranked on a scale from 0 to 100 according to its actual effect on blood sugar levels.

Today we know the G.I. values of hundreds of different food items that have been tested following the standardized method. The complete table of the G.I. values of hundreds of foods can be found in our original book, *The Glucose Revolution* (Marlowe & Company, 1999).

HOW YOU CAN BENEFIT FROM LOW G.I. FOODS

The slow digestion and gradual rise and fall in blood sugar levels after eating low G.I. foods has benefits for many people. Foremost, it helps control blood sugar levels in people with diabetes. It also reduces the secretion of the hormone insulin into the blood (high levels of insulin can increase the risk of heart disease, diabetes and obesity). So low G.I. foods ben-efit people with and without diabetes.

Low G.I. foods:

- cause lower insulin levels that make fat easier to burn and less likely to be stored
- help to lower blood fats
- are more satisfying and reduce appetite
- reduce our risk of developing diabetes and heart disease

These facts are not an exaggeration. They are con-firmed results of studies published in prestigious journals by scientists around the world.

INCLUDING LOW G.I FOODS IN YOUR DIET

Getting the benefits of low G.I. foods is easy—there's nothing complicated about it. All that's required is making a few substitutions like those shown on pages 5–6. Ideally, aim to swap at least half the foods you eat from a high G.I. to a low G.I. type. You might even want to change the type of bread or breakfast cereal and eat pasta or legumes more often.

Using any of the foods in this book will help you to lower the glycemic index of your diet, but it isn't necessary to eat these foods alone. Normally, meals consist of a variety of foods, and we know that eat-ing a low G.I. food with a high G.I. food produces an intermediate G.I. value. Here are three guidelines to help make it easier to include low G.I. foods in your diet:

- become familiar with the choices we list in this book,
- keep them available in your kitchen cupboard (write a shopping list), and
- experiment with them (try new foods and recipes and enjoy what you eat).

■

A HEALTHY, BALANCED DIET CONTAINS A WIDE VARIETY OF LOW FAT, HIGH CARBOHYDRATE FOODS.

■

LOW G.I. SUBSTITUTES

Making the switch to a low G.I. way of eating is simple. Just follow the guidelines below.

SWITCH FROM *THIS* HIGH G.I. FOOD	TO *THIS* LOW G.I. ALTERNATIVE
Bread, whole wheat or white	Breads such as stoneground whole wheat, sourdough and pumpernickel
Processed breakfast cereal	Unrefined cereal such as old-fashioned oats or muesli or a low G.I. processed cereal such as All-Bran Bran Buds with Psyllium™ or All-Bran with extra fiber™
Plain cookies and crackers	Cookies made with dried fruit and whole grains such as oats

Cakes and muffins	These baked goods made with fruit, oats and whole grains
Tropical fruits such as bananas	Temperate climate fruits such as apples, peaches and citrus
Potato	New potatoes, sweet potatoes, corn, pasta and legumes
Rice	Basmati, or Uncle Ben's Converted™, brown or long grain rice

---

STARCH AND THE GLYCEMIC INDEX

Starch granules are composed of two types of starch molecule—a highly branched form called *amylopectin* and a straight chain form called *amylose*. The ratio of the two types of starch in the granule vary from one variety of food to another, and is genetically determined. Different varieties of corn and rice, for example, have different ratios of amylose to amylopectin.

Food processing alters starch granules, making them more readily digested. Manufacturers usually alter the granules by heating them in water (gelatinization), but they may also grind them for the desired effect. During cooking, heat and water make the starch granules swell so that the compact crystalline structure is destroyed. When making gravy with flour and water, the gradual thickening of the mixture corresponds to starch gelatinization. Starches with higher amylose content swell more slowly and at higher temperatures because of stronger binding forces within the granules. In the case of very high amylose starches (such as we find in legumes and high amylose rices), much of the amylose remains ungelatinized at the end of cooking and processing. As a result, there is restricted access by the digestive enzymes, which delays overall digestion and absorption. In general, foods with a high ratio of amylose to amylopectin have lower G.I. values.

LOW G.I. EATING

Low G.I. eating means making a move back to the high carbohydrate foods that are staples in many parts of the world. The emphasis is on whole foods like whole grains—barley, oats, dried peas and beans; in combination with certain types of breads, pasta, rice, vegetables and fruits. Stock your pantry with these foods and keep a loaf of whole grain bread in the freezer. For recipes, check out our book, *The Glucose Revolution* (Marlowe & Co., 1999), which includes more than 60 recipes specially modified to lower the glycemic index, plus new ways of preparing low G.I. foods.

MEASURING THE GLYCEMIC INDEX

Scientists use just six steps to determine the glycemic index of a food. Simple as this may sound, it's actually quite a time-consuming process. Here's how it works.

1. Scientists ask a volunteer to eat an amount of food that contains 50 grams of carbohydrate. For example, to test boiled spaghetti, the volunteer would be given 200 grams of spaghetti, which supplies 50 grams of carbohydrate (we work this out from food composition tables)—50 grams of carbohydrate is equivalent to 3 tablespoons of pure glucose powder.

2. Over the next two hours (or three hours if the volunteer has diabetes), we take a sample of their blood every 15 minutes during the first hour and thereafter every 30 minutes. The blood sugar level of these blood samples is measured in the laboratory and recorded.

3. The blood sugar level is plotted on a graph and the area under the curve is calculated using a computer program (Figure 1).

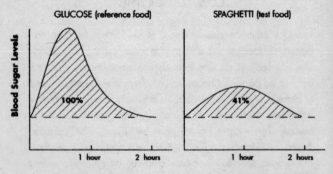

Figure 1. Measuring the glycemic index of a food. The effect of a food on blood sugar levels is calculated using the area under the curve (shaded area). The area under the curve after consumption of the test food is compared with the same area after the reference food (usually 50 grams of pure glucose or a 50 gram carbohydrate portion of white bread).

4. The volunteer's response to spaghetti (or whatever food is being tested) is compared with his or her blood sugar response to 50 grams of pure glucose (the reference food).

5. The reference food is tested on two or three separate occasions and from that we calculate an average value. We do this to reduce the effect of day-to-day variation in blood sugar responses.

6. The average glycemic index found in 8 to 10 people is the glycemic index of that food.

5 KEY FACTORS THAT INFLUENCE
THE GLYCEMIC INDEX

Cooking methods

Cooking and processing increases the glycemic index of a food because it increases the amount of gelatinized starch in the food. Cornflakes is one example.

Physical form of the food

An intact fibrous coat, such as that on grains and legumes, acts as a physical barrier and slows down digestion, lowering a food's glycemic index.

Type of starch

There are two types of starch in foods, amylose and amylopectin. The more amylose starch a food contains, the lower the glycemic index.

Fiber

Viscous, soluble fibers, such as those found in rolled oats and apples, slow down digestion and lower a food's glycemic index.

Sugar

The presence of sugar, as well as the type of sugar, will influence a food's glycemic index. Fruits with a low glycemic index, such as apples and oranges, are high in fructose.

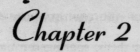

Chapter 2

SOURCES OF CARBOHYDRATE

*C*arbohydrate mainly comes from plant foods, such as cereal grains, fruits, vegetables and legumes (peas and beans). Milk products also contain carbohydrate in the form of milk sugar or lactose, which is the first carbohydrate we eat as infants. Some foods contain a large amount of carbohydrate (cereals, potatoes, legumes are good examples), while other foods, such as carrots, broccoli and salad vegetables are very dilute sources. The dilute sources can be eaten freely, but they won't provide anywhere near enough carbohydrate for our high carbohydrate diet. As nutritious as they can be, salads aren't meals and should be complemented by a carbohydrate-dense food such as bread. The following list includes foods that are high in carbohydrate and provide very little fat. Eat lots of them, sparing the butter, margarine and oil during their preparation.

UNLIMITED VEGETABLES

You can eat most vegetables without thinking about their glycemic index. Most are so low in carbohydrate that they have no measurable effect on our blood sugar levels but they still provide valuable amounts of fiber, vitamins and minerals. Higher carbohydrate vegetables include potato, sweet potato and corn. Among these, corn and sweet potato are the lower G.I. choices. Pumpkin, carrots, peas and beets contain some carbohydrate but a normal serving size contains so little that it does not raise our blood sugar levels significantly.

Salad vegetables such as tomatoes, lettuce, cucumber, peppers and onions have so little carbohydrate that it's impossible to test their glycemic index values. In generous serving sizes, they will have no effect on blood sugars. Think of them as "free" foods that are full of healthful micronutrients. Eat and enjoy!

The best low fat, high carbohydrate choices are:

Cereal grains. These include rice, wheat, oats, barley, rye and anything made from them (bread, pasta, breakfast cereal and flour).

Fruits. A few tasty examples include apples, oranges, bananas, grapes, peaches and melons.

Vegetables. Foods such as potatoes, yams, corn, taro and sweet potato help to create filling, satisfying meals.

Legumes, peas and beans. Baked beans, lentils, kidney beans and chickpeas are a few good choices.

Milk. Not only is milk an excellent source of carbohydrate, it's also rich in bone-building calcium. (Adults should use low fat or skim milk and yogurt to minimize fat intake.)

SOURCES OF CARBOHYDRATE

Percentage of carbohydrate (grams per 3½ ounces of food) in food as eaten

apple	12%
baked beans	11%
banana	21%
barley	61%
bread	47%
cookie	62%
corn	16%
cornflakes	85%
flour	73%
grapes	15%
ice cream	22%
milk	5%
oats	61%
orange	8%
pasta	70%
peas	8%
pear	12%
plum	6%
potato	15–20%
raisins	75%
rice	79%
split peas	45%
sugar	100%
sweet potato	17%
water cracker	71%

THE SUGAR–FAT SEESAW

Did you know that fat and sugar tend to show a reciprocal or seesaw relationship in the diet? Research shows that diets high in fat are low in sugar, and diets low in fat are high in sugar. But studies over the past decade have found that diets high in sugar are no less nutritious than low sugar diets. This is because restricting sugar is frequently followed by higher fat consumption, and most fatty foods are poor sources of nutrients.

In some cases, high sugar diets have been found to have higher micronutrient contents. This is because sugar is often used to sweeten some very nutritious foods, such as yogurts, breakfast cereals and milk.

A low sugar (and high fat) diet has more proven disadvantages than a high sugar (and low fat) diet.

Chapter 3

SECRETS TO LOW G.I. SNACKING

*B*efore we run down the Top 100 foods for you, this might be a good time to talk about snacking. The fact is, low G.I. eating isn't limited to mealtime: It's normal to get hungry and want to snack between your usual "three squares." Luckily, when you eat the low G.I. way there's no prohibition on between-meal nibbles. (It's important to remember that when you choose a snack, glycemic index isn't all that matters; for added health benefits, you should choose a snack that's low in fat, too.)

New evidence suggests that the people who graze, eating small amounts of food throughout the day at frequent intervals, may actually be doing themselves a favor. Spreading the food out over longer periods of time will flatten out the peaks and valleys of blood glucose levels.

ARE YOU REALLY CHOOSING LOW FAT?

There's a trick to food labels that it is worth being aware of when shopping for low fat foods. These food labeling specifications guidelines were enacted by the United States Department of Agriculture (USDA) in 1994:

Free: Contains a tiny or insignificant amount of fat, cholesterol, sodium, sugar or calories: less than 0.5 grams (g) of fat per serving.
Low fat: Contains no more than 3 g of fat per serving.
Reduced/Less/Fewer: These diet products must contain 25 percent less of a nutrient to calories than the regular product.
Light/Lite: These diet products contain ⅓ fewer calories than, or ½ the fat of, the original product.
Lean: Meats with "lean" on the label contain less than 10 g of fat, 4 g of saturated fat, and 95 milligrams (mg) of cholesterol per serving.
Extra lean: These meats have less than 5 g of fat, 2 g of saturated fat and 95 mg of cholesterol per serving.

---

17 SUSTAINING SNACKS

- An apple
- An apple and oat bran muffin
- Dried apricots
- A mini can of baked beans
- A small bowl of cherries
- Ice cream (low fat) in a cone

- Milk, milkshake or smoothie (low fat, of course)
- Oatmeal cookies, 2 to 3
- An orange
- 6 ounces of orange juice, freshly squeezed
- Pita bread spread with apple butter
- A big bowl of low fat popcorn
- 1 or 2 slices of raisin toast
- Whole grain bread sandwich with your favorite filling
- A bowl of oatmeal
- A small box of raisins
- 6 to 8 ounces of light yogurt

6 SNACKING TIPS

- It is important to include a couple of servings of dairy foods each day to meet your calcium needs. If you haven't used yogurt or cheese in any meals, you may choose to make a low fat milkshake. One or 2 scoops of low fat ice cream or pudding can also boost your daily calcium intake.
- If you like whole grain breads, an extra slice makes a very good choice for a snack. Other snacks can include toasted sourdough English muffin halves, a waffle or a slice of raisin bread with a little butter.
- Fruit is always a low calorie option for snacks. You should try to consume *at least* 3 servings a day. It may be helpful to prepare fruit in advance to make it accessible and easy to eat.
- Ryvita whole grain crispbreads are a low calorie snack if you want something dry and crunchy.

- Popcorn is another crunchy snack choice. You can make your own air popped treat (using a minimum of oil), or try a microwaved version such as the brand listed on page 103.
- Keep vegetables (such as celery and carrot sticks, baby tomatoes, florets of blanched cauliflower or broccoli) ready prepared.

Chapter 4

LOW G.I. FOODS BY CATEGORY

BREAD

Chapati (Baisen)

GLYCEMIC INDEX: 27

■

1 4-ounce chapati contains:

CARBOHYDRATE:	44 g
FAT:	1 g (made without oil)
FIBER:	3 g

Chapati is an unleavened or slightly leavened Indian bread, which resembles pita bread in appearance. Though it's often made with wheat flour, it is also made from *baisen*, or chick pea flour, which is milled from a small variety of chickpeas. Chapati made from baisen has a significantly lower glycemic index than that made from wheat flour, due to the nature of the starch. All legumes, including chickpeas, have a higher proportion of amylose starch than found in cereal grains.

To date, researchers have measured the glycemic index of only a few nationally available breads. And although it's impossible to know for certain without testing products individually, other heavy grain breads not listed here may have similar low G.I. values.

Natural Ovens
100% Whole Grain Bread

GLYCEMIC INDEX: 51

■

1 slice of this whole grain bread contains:

CARBOHYDRATE:	17 g
FAT:	less than 1 g
FIBER:	5 g

This loaf is one of the Natural Ovens's highest fiber breads, boasting 5 grams of fiber per slice. This bread is a pure, whole grain, low fat loaf. The company uses stoneground whole wheat flour, which produces larger carbohydrate particle sizes (whereas high G.I. white bread has very small easily digested carbohydrate particles). This bread also contains oats, a source of soluble fiber, and is fortified with lots of additional fiber, too. Natural Ovens breads are available in the United States by mail order. For ordering information, see page 121.

Natural Ovens Happiness Bread

GLYCEMIC INDEX: 63

■

1 slice of Happiness bread contains:

CARBOHYDRATE:	15 g
FAT:	0 g
FIBER:	5 g

With its added raisins, pecans and cinnamon, Happiness Bread is so good many people enjoy it for dessert! The company uses stoneground whole wheat flour, which produces larger carbohydrate particle sizes. The oats provide a source of soluble fiber, and the raisins and fructose both serve as low G.I. sweeteners. That, along with the relatively slow fermentation time, help to make this a filling low G.I. bread. Natural Ovens breads are available in the United States by mail order. For ordering information, see page 121.

Natural Ovens Hunger Filler Bread

GLYCEMIC INDEX: 59

■

1 slice of Hunger Filler bread contains:

CARBOHYDRATE:	16 g
FAT:	less than 1 g
FIBER:	5 g

Hunger Filler Bread is so filling that it keeps you satisfied from meal to meal—great for weight-watchers! This loaf contains ½ gram of fat per serving, and is loaded with fiber from wheat bran, wheat germ, oat bran, flaxseed and sesame seeds. Hunger Filler Bread uses stoneground whole wheat flour and contains oat and rice bran (soluble fiber) and fructose. A relatively slow fermentation time (three rising periods) contributes to its low glycemic index. Natural Ovens breads are available in the United States by mail order. For ordering information, see page 121.

Natural Ovens Natural Wheat Bread

GLYCEMIC INDEX: 59

■

1 slice of Natural Wheat Bread contains:

CARBOHYDRATE:	16 g
FAT:	less than 1 g
FIBER:	5 g

This loaf contains 5 grams of fiber per slice, making it a whole grain, low fat loaf. The company uses whole wheat flour, which produces larger carbohydrate particles and contains steel cut oats, a source of soluble fiber, and cracked wheat as well as fructose (a low G.I. sugar). The bread's three rising periods and relatively slow fermentation time contribute to its low glycemic index. Natural Ovens breads are available in the United States by mail order. For ordering information, see page 121.

Pita, Whole Wheat

GLYCEMIC INDEX: 57

■

1 2-ounce pita bread
(approximately 6 inches in diameter) contains:

CARBOHYDRATE:	35 g
FAT:	2 g
FIBER:	4 g

Researchers have found that flat bread such as pita has a lower glycemic index than regular bread. Pita bread has become a popular prepackaged bread item in most supermarkets and grocery stores. You can toast it, stuff it or dress it like a pizza! The lower glycemic index may result from a denser molecular structure that resists digestion in the small intestine compared with the light airy texture of regular bread.

Pumpernickel Bread

GLYCEMIC INDEX: 51

■

1 slice of pumpernickel bread contains:

CARBOHYDRATE:	15 g
FAT:	1 g
FIBER:	3 g

Also known as rye kernel bread, pumpernickel contains 80 to 90 percent whole and cracked rye kernels. It has a strong flavor and is dense and compact—not "airy" as some breads are. Pumpernickel is usually sold thinly sliced. The main reason for its low glycemic index is its content of whole cereal grains. (Bread made from whole wheat grains would be expected to have a similarly low glycemic index.)

Rye Bread

GLYCEMIC INDEX: 65

■

1 slice of rye (1 ounce) bread contains:

CARBOHYDRATE:	15 g
FAT:	1 g
FIBER:	2 g

Bakers use rye flour extensively when making bread. Because its protein (gluten) is not very elastic, the dough doesn't trap as much gas as it leavens, giving rye bread its characteristic dense, compact look. It is difficult to separate the germ and bran layers in the milling process of rye grains into flour. Dark rye flour contains several B vitamins as well as such minerals as magnesium, potassium, zinc phosphorus, iron, copper and calcium.

Sourdough Bread

GLYCEMIC INDEX: 52

■

1 1½-ounce slice of sourdough bread contains:

CARBOHYDRATE:	20 g
FAT:	1 g
FIBER:	1 g

Sourdough results from the deliberately slow fermentation of flour by yeast, which produces a buildup of organic acids. These acids give the bread its characteristic sour taste. Once it's eaten, sourdough bread is slowly released from the stomach into the small intestine, where the body digests it. The slower the rate of "gastric emptying," the slower the conversion into glucose into the blood. This is why sourdough breads have low G.I. values.

Sourdough Rye Bread (Arnold's)

GLYCEMIC INDEX: 57

■

1 1½-ounce slice of sourdough rye contains:

CARBOHYDRATE:	21 g
FAT:	1 g
FIBER:	less than 1 g

A buildup of organic acids give sourdough bread its characteristic sour taste. This flavorful low G.I. bread is a popular choice for take out sandwiches to the office or for picnics or travel, because its compact structure keeps the sandwich intact. And the sour flavor blends well with a wide variety of cold cut sandwich fillers.

Stoneground Whole Wheat Bread

GLYCEMIC INDEX: 53

■

*1 1-ounce slice of stoneground
whole wheat bread contains:*

CARBOHYDRATE:	15 g
FAT:	1 g
FIBER:	2 g

"Stoneground 100% whole wheat bread" means that the flour used has been milled from the entire wheat berry (the germ, endosperm or starch compartment and the bran) and that the milling process used is a method of slowly grinding the grain with a buhrstone instead of metal rollers to more evenly distribute the germ oil. Virtually none of the ingredients packaged in the wheat berry gets lost in this processing method. This bread is a rich source of several B vitamins, iron, zinc and dietary fiber.

BREAKFAST CEREALS

All-Bran Bran Buds with Psyllium ™ (Kellogg's)

GLYCEMIC INDEX: 45

■

⅓ cup of Bran Buds contains:

CARBOHYDRATE:	24 g
FAT:	1 g
FIBER:	13 g

Along with All-Bran with extra fiber, All-Bran Bran Buds are the most fiber-rich breakfast cereals. The sources of fiber come from wheat and corn bran and psyllium (a soluble fiber that helps to reduce the risk of heart disease). This is a low G.I. food that, because it is digested so slowly, keeps you feeling full for hours. Combine it with skim or 1% milk and fresh or unsweetened canned fruit for a great start to your day.

All-Bran With Extra Fiber ™ (Kellogg's)

GLYCEMIC INDEX: 51

■

½ cup of All-Bran with extra fiber contains:

CARBOHYDRATE:	20 g
FAT:	1 g
FIBER:	13 g

This cereal is a good source of B vitamins, as well as an excellent source of insoluble fiber. All-Bran is made from coarsely milled wheat bran that has large pieces of endosperm (starch) still attached. This minimizes the swelling of the starch molecules and limits the action of the digestive enzymes.

All-Bran with extra fiber has a malty taste and is good topped with fresh or unsweetened canned fruit slices and milk. Alternatively, sprinkle a few tablespoons over a lower fiber cereal to help meet your daily fiber requirement. All-Bran with extra fiber can also be added to muffins where it will boost the fiber content and lower the glycemic index of the finished product.

Cream of Wheat, Old Fashioned

GLYCEMIC INDEX: 66

■

¼ cup cooked Cream of Wheat contains:

CARBOHYDRATE:	21 g
FAT:	0 g
FIBER:	less than 1 g

Cream of Wheat is a cooked hot cereal served by itself or with fruit, sugar or cinnamon. Its ingredients, whole meal wheat (or farina) and wheat germ, explain this breakfast food's relatively low glycemic index. It provides an excellent source of iron and a good source of calcium—all for a minimum of fat and calories.

Muesli, Natural

GLYCEMIC INDEX: 56

■

⅓ cup (1½ ounces) of natural muesli contains:

CARBOHYDRATE:	28 g
FAT:	3 g
FIBER:	5 g

Muesli originated as a Swiss health food and nowadays rates as one of the few relatively unprocessed breakfast cereals on the market. It is a good source of carbohydrate, thiamin, riboflavin and niacin. The low glycemic index results because the oats are eaten raw, and are therefore in an ungelatinized state that resists digestion in the small intestine. Oats also contain a fiber that increases the viscosity of the contents of the small intestine, thereby slowing down the enzyme attack. This same fiber has also been shown to reduce blood cholesterol levels.

Muesli, Breakfast Cereal, Toasted

GLYCEMIC INDEX: 43

■

2/3 cup (2 ounces) contains:

CARBOHYDRATE:	41 g
FAT:	3 g
FIBER:	4 g

Some commercial brands of toasted muesli have large quantities of added fat. Although the fat may help to lower the food's glycemic index, it also grossly increases the number of calories you're eating. You can find healthier versions of these mueslis in some health food stores (they may use monounsaturated oils to toast the grains) or in mail order catalogs. You can also search the Web for whole-food companies that may produce lower fat muesli. Better yet, why not develop your own recipe?

Multi-Bran Chex ™ (General Mills)

GLYCEMIC INDEX: 58

■

1 cup (2 ounces) of Multi-Bran Chex contains:

CARBOHYDRATE:	49 g
FAT:	2 g
FIBER:	7 g

The high fiber content in this cereal comes from a mixture of wheat, rice and corn brans. If you eat it as a breakfast cereal, Multi-Bran Chex is a low fat, high fiber, relatively low G.I. food. The calcium already in the cereal, plus the milk added on top, provides another nutrient bonus. You can also use Multi-Bran Chex to make a healthy snack mix with dried fruit and nuts.

Oat Bran Breakfast Cereal™ (Quaker Oats)

GLYCEMIC INDEX: 50

∎

¾ cup (1 ounce) contains:

CARBOHYDRATE:	23 g
FAT:	1 g
FIBER:	4 g

Quaker Oats oat bran breakfast cereal is just like the hot bran cereal except that it contains dry flakes of natural oat bran and whole grain wheat. The oat bran contains soluble fiber, which is believed to lower cholesterol and reduce the risk of heart disease when included as part of a high fiber low fat diet. Add fresh or natural canned fruit and skim or 1% milk and you'll start your day with an energy packed and nutritionally dense breakfast.

Oatmeal, Old Fashioned

GLYCEMIC INDEX: 49

■

½ cup cooked old fashioned oatmeal contains:

CARBOHYDRATE:	12 g
FAT:	1 g
FIBER:	4 g

Old fashioned cooked oats are a good source of viscous soluble fiber, B vitamins, vitamin E, iron and zinc. Rolled oats are hulled, steamed and flattened, which makes oatmeal a 100% whole grain cereal. The additional flaking of rolled oats to produce quick cooking oats increases the rate of digestion, which results in a higher glycemic index. This is why *old fashioned* oats are preferred over quick or instant. Supplementing a low fat diet with rolled oats can help to lower your cholesterol. Don't be afraid to add a little brown sugar and milk to increase your enjoyment of this healthy cooked cereal.

Shredded Wheat ™ (Post)

GLYCEMIC INDEX: 58

■

⅔ cup of spoonsize Shredded Wheat contains:

CARBOHYDRATE:	27 g
FAT:	0 g
FIBER:	3 g

Shredded Wheat is one of very few commercially prepared cereals that contains absolutely no additives:
Its one and only ingredient is 100 percent natural
whole wheat. The intact fibrous structure of the cereal gives it its low glycemic index. To add extra flavor,
you can top Shredded Wheat with cinnamon, sugar
or fresh or unsweetened canned fruit.

$\mathcal{S}pecial\,\mathcal{K}^{TM}\,(\mathcal{K}ellogg's)$

GLYCEMIC INDEX: 54

■

1 cup of Special K contains:

CARBOHYDRATE:	22 g
FAT:	0 g
FIBER:	1 g

Special K has twice the protein content (20 percent) of normal breakfast cereals. The high protein slows down the rate of stomach emptying, which reduces the rate of starch digestion and absorption. Topped with low fat or skim milk and topped with fresh or unsweetened canned fruit, a bowl of Special K™ cereal can leave you feeling full for hours after breakfast.

CEREAL GRAINS

Barley, Pearled

GLYCEMIC INDEX: 25

■

½ cup of pearled barley, boiled, contains:

CARBOHYDRATE:	22 g
FAT:	0 g
FIBER:	3 g

Pearled barley, a popular form of this cereal grain, has had the outer brown layers of husk removed. It is very nutritious and high in fiber with one of the lowest G.I. values of any food. Much of the fiber is a viscous, soluble fiber, which helps to reduce the post-meal rise in blood glucose. It does this by slowing down the movement of the partially digested food through the small intestine, which slows down digestion. The near intact structure of the grain also keeps the glycemic index low. Use it as you would rice; you can also add it to soups and stews.

Buckwheat Groats (Kasha)

GLYCEMIC INDEX: 54 (AVERAGE)

■

*½ cup of roasted buckwheat groats,
cooked, contains:*

CARBOHYDRATE:	20 g
FAT:	1 g
FIBER:	3 g

Buckwheat grains must be hulled to be edible. The cracked whole buckwheat "groats" that result from hulling can be roasted and used just like rice or potatoes in soups, pilafs or stews, or as a cooked cereal. People also use buckwheat flour in pancakes, muffins, cookies and cakes and to make Russian "blinis" and Japanese "soba" noodles. In any form, buckwheat is a source of potassium, magnesium, zinc, iron, calcium, copper and several of the B vitamins. They also provide soluble fiber.

Bulgur (Cracked Wheat)

GLYCEMIC INDEX: 48

■

⅓ cup of bulgur, boiled, contains:

CARBOHYDRATE:	23 g
FAT:	0 g
FIBER:	8 g

Bulgur is made by coarsely grinding dried cooked wheat grains. The parboiling and light crushing of the wheat grain in the process of making bulgur has only a small effect on the glycemic index. This grain is popular in Middle Eastern cuisine: Bulgur is most commonly recognized as the main ingredient in Lebanese "tabouli," a mixture of parsley, bulgur, chopped tomato, onion and dressing. The compactness and intact physical form of the wheat contributes to its low glycemic index.

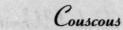

Couscous

GLYCEMIC INDEX: 65

■

⅔ cup couscous, cooked, contains:

CARBOHYDRATE:	21 g
FAT:	0 g
FIBER:	1 g

Coarsely ground semolina, a hard-wheat flour used for making pasta, is the main ingredient in couscous. Technically a pasta, couscous is interchangeable with rice, bulgur and other small grains in soups and salads. You can use it in pilafs, desserts or as a hot cereal, or use it as an accompaniment to meat and vegetable dishes. It's also great topped with spicy curry sauces.

Oat Bran, Raw

GLYCEMIC INDEX: 55

■

1 tablespoon of raw oat bran contains:

CARBOHYDRATE:	7 g
FAT:	1 g
FIBER:	2 g

Unprocessed oat bran is available in the cereal section of supermarkets. Its carbohydrate content is lower than that of oats and it is higher in fiber, particularly soluble fiber, which is responsible for its low glycemic index. When mixed with water, oat bran forms a jelly-like mixture that increases the viscosity of the solution in the small intestine. This slows down the movement of enzymes and food, resulting in slower digestion. A soft, bland product, oat bran is a useful addition to breakfast cereals and as a partial substitution for flour in baked goods to help lower the food's glycemic index.

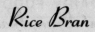

Rice Bran

GLYCEMIC INDEX: 19

■

1 tablespoon of rice bran contains:

CARBOHYDRATE:	5 g
FAT:	2 g
FIBER:	2 g

Rice bran is a good source of thiamin, riboflavin and niacin and has a sweet malty flavor. Rice bran is actually the outer bran layer that is scraped from brown rice in the milling of white rice, and it contains the fibrous seed coat and a small part of the germ. It is rich in fiber (25 percent by weight) and oil (20 percent by weight) and has an extremely low glycemic index. Rice bran is available in the cereal section of supermarkets. Sprinkle it on breakfast cereal or add to baked goods or meatloaf.

DAIRY FOODS

Ice Cream (Low Fat)

GLYCEMIC INDEX: 50

■

½ cup (2 ounces) of reduced-fat ice cream contains:

CARBOHYDRATE:	15 g
FAT:	3 g
FIBER:	0 g

Ice cream is a source of calcium. Look for low fat or nonfat ice creams when you shop. Some taste as good or better than their full fat counterparts! Ice cream has a higher glycemic index than milk alone because of the presence of sucrose and glucose in addition to lactose. The mixture of low and high G.I. sugars leads to an intermediate G.I. food.

Milk, Chocolate, 1% Milk Fat

GLYCEMIC INDEX: 34

■

1 cup (8 ounces) 1% chocolate milk contains:

CARBOHYDRATE:	26 g
FAT:	3 g
FIBER:	1 g

Adding a moderate amount of refined sugar in the form of chocolate syrup or powder does not significantly raise the glycemic index of 1% milk. For many young people (and adults as well) who don't care for the taste of plain milk or prefer something a bit sweeter, this is an excellent dairy choice that can help add some extra vitamins and minerals to the day's nutrient intake.

Milk, Skim

GLYCEMIC INDEX: 32

■

1 cup (8 ounces) of skim milk contains:

CARBOHYDRATE:	12 g
FAT:	0 g
FIBER:	0 g

This is the most nutritious form of milk for the least amount of calories (approximately 90). The glycemic index of skim milk is only slightly higher than that of whole milk, because there is no fat to slow down the gastric emptying. But all forms of milk are low G.I. foods. For people trying to cut fat in their diet, switching from whole or low fat milk to skim is a great first step.

Milk, Whole

GLYCEMIC INDEX: 27 (AVERAGE)

■

1 cup (8 ounces) of whole milk contains:

CARBOHYDRATE:	11 g
FAT:	9 g
FIBER:	0 g

Milk is a rich source of protein and vitamin B_2 (riboflavin). Unfortunately, whole milk is also a rich source of saturated fat and cholesterol, so it's healthier to consume low fat and nonfat milk and milk products instead. The surprisingly low glycemic index of milk is a result of two factors that lessen its glycemic effect. First, lactose, the primary sugar in milk, breaks down into glucose and galactose. Within our bodies, these two simple sugars compete for, and slow down each other's absorption. Additionally, the milk protein forms a soft curd in the stomach and slows down the rate of stomach emptying. People who are lactose intolerant can find lactose-reduced milks on supermarket shelves.

Hot milk and honey makes a nutritious nightcap. Research shows that people do indeed sleep sounder after drinking milk at night. The active component is an amino acid called tryptophan, which the body converts to serotonin—the neurotransmitter associated with calmness and well-being.

Yogurt, Nonfat, Fruit Flavored, with Artificial Sweetener

GLYCEMIC INDEX: 14

■

8 ounces of nonfat yogurt contains:

CARBOHYDRATE:	16 g
FAT:	0 g
FIBER:	0 g

All varieties of yogurt have low glycemic index values. When sweetened artificially, flavored yogurt has an even lower glycemic index and contains fewer calories than naturally sweetened yogurt. You can eat fruited yogurts right out of the container for a quick snack or meal addition, or you can mix it with a few tablespoons of low G.I. cereal for a heartier snack.

Yogurt, Nonfat, Fruit Flavored, with Sugar

GLYCEMIC INDEX: 33

■

8 ounces of nonfat yogurt contains:

CARBOHYDRATE:	30 g
FAT:	0 g
FIBER:	0 g

When yogurt is made, the bacterial culture added to milk breaks down some of the lactose into lactic acid, which denatures the protein and forms a soft curd. The acidity and high protein content slow down stomach emptying contributing to the low G.I. value. In fruit yogurts (G.I. = 33), the addition of sugar sweetened fruit syrup mixtures increases their glycemic index over that of an artificially sweetened yogurt (G.I. = 14). Lactose intolerant people can safely consume yogurt containing live cultures without fear of symptoms.

Yogurt, Nonfat, Plain

GLYCEMIC INDEX: 14

■

8 ounces of nonfat yogurt contains:

CARBOHYDRATE:	17 g
FAT:	0 g
FIBER:	0 g

Nonfat plain yogurt has the highest nutrient density and the fewest calories of all forms of yogurt: It's an excellent source of protein, calcium, phosphorus, potassium and vitamins A and B. A concentrated milk product, yogurt taste is soured by the use of specific bacteria. As with milk, yogurt contains lactose, a sugar that breaks down into glucose and galactose. Within our bodies these two simple sugars compete with each other for absorption. The bacterial cultures in yogurt convert some of the sugar in milk (lactose) into lactic acid, making it more acidic. Yogurt contains a considerable amount of protein (8g/8 ozs.), not all of which the body breaks down into glucose. For these three reasons—the presence of the simple sugar galactose, its low acidity, and its high protein content—yogurt has a very low glycemic index value.

FRUIT AND FRUIT JUICES

Apple Juice

GLYCEMIC INDEX: 40

■

1 cup (8 ounces) of unsweetened apple juice contains:

CARBOHYDRATE:	29 g
FAT:	0 g
FIBER:	0 g

Apple juice has a low glycemic index because of its high fructose content. Apples in all forms—and colors!—contain potassium and vitamin C. Apple juice has some diuretic and laxative properties and aids in the overall functioning of the digestive system.

Apple, Dried

GLYCEMIC INDEX: 29

∎

1 ounce of dried apple (about 5 rings) contains:

CARBOHYDRATE:	24 g
FAT:	0 g
FIBER:	3 g

Dried fruits, such as dried apples, are currently gaining popularity with consumers. They are a convenient and healthy snack food, as well as tasty ingredients in granolas, trail mixes and baked fruit bars. They are available with or without added sugar, sulfured or unsulfured and even in organic varieties. The nutritive value of dried apples is obviously elevated in comparison to the fresh fruit when compared by weight. So even just a few dried apple rings can provide lots of vitamins and minerals to your diet. Dried apples are a good source of potassium, vitamin C and soluble and insoluble fiber.

Apple, Fresh

GLYCEMIC INDEX: 38

■

1 medium sized apple (about 5 ounces) contains:

CARBOHYDRATE:	18 g
FAT:	0 g
FIBER:	4 g

Apples provide a crunchy, portable low G.I. snack that's also a good source of fiber. Half the sugar in apples is fructose, which has a very low glycemic index. Fructose is more slowly absorbed than glucose and is only gradually converted to glucose in the liver. Apples are also high in malic acid (all acids slow down stomach emptying) and pectin (a soluble and viscous fiber that slows down the digestive process by increasing the viscosity of the intestinal contents). All these factors act together to make apples a low G.I. food.

Whole apples cause less secretion of the hormone insulin than apple puree or juice, but the reasons, so far, are not entirely clear. Despite this, apple juice has a glycemic index very close to whole apples. Cooking apples is likely to raise the glycemic index slightly because it breaks down the cell wall.

Apricot, Dried

GLYCEMIC INDEX: 31

■

5 dried apricot halves contain:

CARBOHYDRATE:	13 g
FAT:	0 g
FIBER:	2 g

Dried apricots provide an excellent source of fiber and beta-carotene (the plant precursor of vitamin A) and are also a source of iron. This dried fruit makes a nourishing snack or addition to a school lunch box. The chewy compact structure of dried apricots probably limits access by digestive juices and explains the reduction in glycemic index compared with fresh apricots. Half the sugars are in the form of fructose, which produces very little effect on blood sugar levels.

Apricot, Fresh

GLYCEMIC INDEX: 57

■

3 medium apricots contain:

CARBOHYDRATE:	12 g
FAT:	0 g
FIBER:	3 g

Like apples, apricots are high in fructose (about half their carbohydrate), which contributes to their low glycemic index. Apricots are known for their very high vitamin A content; they are also rich in potassium and vitamin C. Apricots can help stimulate a depressed appetite. As with all orange-yellow plant foods, apricots are good sources of several antioxidant vitamins.

Cherries

GLYCEMIC INDEX: 22

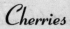

10 large cherries (fresh or raw) contain:

CARBOHYDRATE:	10 g
FAT:	0 g
FIBER:	2 g

Cherries are a good source of potassium and vitamin C and have the lowest glycemic index of any fruit scientists have examined so far. We don't know exactly why the cherry's glycemic index is so low, but this fruit does have a somewhat rubbery consistency, just like pasta and dried apricots, which is known to increase resistance to disruption in the intestine. Cherries are also acidic and high in sugars, both of which slow down the rate of stomach emptying (and therefore digestion). Canned cherries in heavy syrup are likely to have a higher glycemic index. Cherries provide potassium, vitamin A and fiber. This fruit must be picked ripe since they will not ripen after harvesting.

Fruit Cocktail

GLYCEMIC INDEX: 55

■

½ cup of canned fruit cocktail in natural juice contains:

CARBOHYDRATE:	15 g
FAT:	0 g
FIBER:	1 g

Fruit cocktail usually consists of a mixture of peaches, pears, seedless grapes, pineapple and cherries—mostly low G.I. fruit! In fact, the majority of fruits have a low G.I; the presence of sugars (especially fructose), which have low G.I. values, fiber (both soluble and insoluble) and acids (which may slow down stomach emptying) are probable reasons. The lowest G.I. fruits tend to be those grown in temperate climates such as apples, pears, citrus and peaches. The more acidic the fruit, the lower the glycemic index (for example, a grapefruit's glycemic index is 25). Tropical fruits like melons, pineapple and bananas have intermediate glycemic index values. All fresh fruits are a source of vitamin C, so try to include several servings in your diet every day. Cans labeled "natural," "lite/light" and "in real fruit juices" are all ways of saying that there has been no sugar added to the canned fruit.

Grapefruit

GLYCEMIC INDEX: 25

■

½ a medium grapefruit contains:

CARBOHYDRATE:	5 g
FAT:	0 g
FIBER:	1 g

Half a grapefruit contains about 42 mg of vitamin C, making it an excellent source for this antioxidant. It is high in citric acid, which lowers the glycemic index by slowing down stomach emptying. Grapefruit is a refreshing food to eat at breakfast, halved and eaten as is or sprinkled with a little sugar. They can also be peeled and segmented and included in fruit or vegetable salads.

Grapefruit Juice

GLYCEMIC INDEX: 48

■

1 cup of unsweetened grapefruit juice contains:

CARBOHYDRATE:	22 g
FAT:	0 g
FIBER:	0 g

Cool and refreshing after a workout or with breakfast, a glass of grapefruit juice provides not only liq-
uid refreshment, but nutritional benefits, as well.
Rich in the antioxidant vitamin C, grapefruit juice is
also high in citric acid, which slows down stomach
emptying and lowers the juice's glycemic index.
Many commercial brands now add extra calcium to
grapefruit juice for a drink that's a powerhouse of
antioxidant and bone-building protection. For a new
taste sensation, try mixing grapefruit juice with club
soda—the result is a tangy, fizzy beverage!

Grapes, Green

GLYCEMIC INDEX: 46

■

1 cup of green grapes contains:

CARBOHYDRATE:	15 g
FAT:	0 g
FIBER:	1 g

Grapes have one of the highest sugar contents among temperate fruits. This is one reason they make a good starting product for alcoholic beverages (more sugar means more alcohol). The high sugar content reduces the rate of stomach emptying, which slows down digestion and absorption. Grapes are also quite high in acid, another factor that slows down the rate of food entering the small intestine. They're the perfect snack food—convenient to carry and eat on the run. No mess!

Kiwi

GLYCEMIC INDEX: 52

■

1 medium kiwi (about 2½ ounces) contains:

CARBOHYDRATE:	8 g
FAT:	0 g
FIBER:	3 g

The furry kiwi provides lots of the antioxidant vitamin C. This acidic fruit contains equal proportions of glucose (high glycemic index) and fructose (low glycemic index), which results in an intermediate G.I. value. Kiwis are also quite acidic; the acids slow down stomach emptying and result in slower rates of digestion and absorption in the small intestine.

Mango

GLYCEMIC INDEX: 55

■

1 small mango (about 5 ounces) contains:

CARBOHYDRATE:	19 g
FAT:	0 g
FIBER:	2 g

Mango is one tropical fruit that squeezes into the low G.I. range. Most tropical fruits have a higher glycemic index than temperate fruit, possibly related to differences in acidity and sugar content. It is rich in naturally occurring sugars, vitamin C and vitamin A precursors. Mangoes are a versatile fruit that you can eat in fruit salads and crepes and as an accompaniment to fish, meat, poultry and legumes. You can also enjoy it with breakfast cereals or all by itself. At its peak ripeness, a mango is sure to please every palate.

Orange, Navel

GLYCEMIC INDEX: 44

■

1 medium orange (approximately 4 ounces) contains:

CARBOHYDRATE:	10 g
FAT:	0 g
FIBER:	3 g

Oranges are major sources of vitamin C. One orange can provide around 60 mg of vitamin C!

Much of the sugar content of oranges is sucrose, a "double" sugar made up of glucose and fructose. When it's digested, only the glucose molecule makes an impression on blood sugar levels. This and orange's high acid content account for their low G.I. value.

Papaya

GLYCEMIC INDEX: 58

∎

½ medium (5 ounces) contains:

CARBOHYDRATE:	14 g
FAT:	0 g
FIBER:	3 g

The papaya is a fruit rich in the antioxidant vitamins A and C, as well as fiber and potassium. Its versatility makes it a perfect choice mixed into yogurt, puddings, frozen desserts, fruit salads, purees and juices. With a mellow flavor similar to melon, papaya goes well with baked ham, prosciutto, smoked salmon, chicken and seafood salads. When buying a papaya, choose one with a skin that's almost completely red-orange that will yield slightly to the touch, which indicates perfect ripeness.

Peach, Canned, Natural Juice

GLYCEMIC INDEX: 30

■

*½ cup (4 ounces) canned peaches in fruit juice con-
tains:*

CARBOHYDRATE:	14 g
FAT:	0 g
FIBER:	2 g

Peaches canned in natural juice have a low glycemic
index perhaps because the final product has a higher
osmolality (osmotic pressure) that slows down stomach emptying. Peaches canned in heavy sugar syrup
have a substantially higher G.I. value (almost double)
because of the addition of refined sugar.

Peach, Fresh

GLYCEMIC INDEX: 42

■

1 medium peach (approximately 3 ounces) contains:

CARBOHYDRATE:	7 g
FAT:	0 g
FIBER:	2 g

Much of the sugar in peaches is sucrose (4.7 percent), which is identical to normal table sugar. It is a "double" sugar made up of glucose and fructose. When digested, only the glucose molecule makes an impression on blood sugar levels. This fact, along with the soluble fiber content and natural acidity account for peaches' low glycemic index. A peach is a good source of vitamins A and C, niacin and potassium. Since peaches are often coated with a thin layer of wax to prolong shelf life, wash them well before eating.

Pear, Canned, Natural Juice

GLYCEMIC INDEX: 44

■

½ cup (4 ounces) canned pears in pear juice contains:

CARBOHYDRATE:	13 g
FAT:	0 g
FIBER:	2 g

The glycemic index of a canned pear is only slightly higher than that of the fresh fruit. This is because fructose, the low G.I. natural sugar found in fruit, remains in high concentration in the pears even when they are canned. Pears are rich in fiber, potassium and copper. Dehydrated or dried pears, now more commonly found in the produce departments of supermarkets, contain an even more concentrated supply of valuable vitamins and minerals.

Pear, Fresh

GLYCEMIC INDEX: 38

■

1 medium pear (approximately 5 ounces) contains:

CARBOHYDRATE:	21 g
FAT:	0 g
FIBER:	4 g

Pears have a high content of fructose (6.7 percent), a sugar that has minimal effect on blood sugars. Pears are at their peak during autumn. They ripen quickly and should be eaten before they get too soft. They are a nice accompaniment to cheese and walnuts on a platter for dessert. They also make a stylish dessert poached or baked in a syrup or red wine.

Plum

GLYCEMIC INDEX: 39

■

1 medium plum (about 2 ounces) contains:

CARBOHYDRATE:	7 g
FAT:	0 g
FIBER:	1 g

The combination of organic acids and high concentration of sugars slows down the rate of stomach emptying, which reduces the glycemic response. Plums also contain viscous fiber, which reduces the rate of digestion in the small intestine. They make a light, tasty snack—just have a napkin nearby to catch the juice!

LEGUMES

Baked Beans

GLYCEMIC INDEX: 48

■

½ cup of vegetarian baked beans in tomato sauce contains:

CARBOHYDRATE:	24 g
FAT:	1 g
FIBER:	6 g

A popular, ready-to-eat form of legumes. The digestibility of legumes is determined primarily by the nature of the starch that's trapped in fibrous, thick-walled cells, which prevents the starch from swelling during cooking, slowing down its digestibility. Baked beans are commonly made from navy beans, which (like all legumes) have a high concentration of amylose.

Home-cooked baked beans have a lower glycemic index (38) than canned baked beans. The process of canning plus the addition of sugar in the sauce raises the glycemic index, but not excessively. Canned baked beans are still a good low G.I. choice and are a healthy addition to any meal.

Black Beans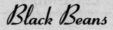

GLYCEMIC INDEX: 30

■

¼ cup (4½ ounces) boiled black beans contains:

CARBOHYDRATE:	31 g
FAT:	0 g
FIBER:	12 g

The black bean is a completely black kidney-shaped small bean used most often in Mexican cooking. It can also be added to soups and salads for extra flavor and texture. As with other legumes, the black bean is a high fiber food that our bodies digest slowly, permitting sustained feelings of fullness for several hours.

Blackeyed Peas

GLYCEMIC INDEX: 42

■

½ cup of black-eyed peas contains:

CARBOHYDRATE:	16 g
FAT:	1 g
FIBER:	5 g

Also known as cowpeas and Southern peas, these are a small, kidney-shaped, creamy colored bean with a distinctive black "eye" and a subtle sweet flavor. Use them for soups and stews and in bean salads. They can be pureed and are a traditional accompaniment to pork in the southern United States. They are an excellent source of folic acid, magnesium and potassium, and a good source of iron, phosphorus and certain B vitamins. They should be cooked for about an hour; be careful not to overcook them or they will turn mushy. Blackeyed peas cause a smaller glucose rise because of the relatively slow or incomplete breakdown of their starch, which is mainly due to containment of the starch in intact cell walls and by its relatively high amylose content. The presence of phenolic compounds (such as tannins and catechins) in legumes tends to slow down digestion by inhibiting the action of the amylase enzymes.

Chana Dal

GLYCEMIC INDEX: 8

■

1 ½-cup serving of chana dal contains:

CARBOHYDRATE:	28 g
FAT:	3 g
FIBER:	8 g

Chana dal, the bean with the lowest glycemic index, is a diet staple in India, but is still little known in the United States. The chana dal bean looks just like a yellow split pea, but when it's cooked, it doesn't readily boil down to mush the way split peas do. It is more closely related to chickpeas (garbanzo beans), but chana dal is younger, smaller and sweeter, with a much lower glycemic index value. In fact, you can substitute chana dal for chickpeas in just about any recipe. You can eat pureed chana dal with rice, or the dry bean with bread. A nutritious form of plant protein, chana dal is an excellent source of folic acid and fiber. Chana dal is generally available in Indian and Southeast Asian food stores. As awareness of the value of eating low G.I. foods spreads, this bean is becoming more widely available. If you don't see it at your favorite food store, ask your local health food store or specialty grocer to carry it.

Chickpeas, Boiled

GLYCEMIC INDEX: 33

■

½ cup boiled chickpeas, drained, contains:

CARBOHYDRATE:	23 g
FAT:	2 g
FIBER:	6 g

A particularly versatile legume that is rich in protein, B vitamins and minerals, chickpeas are the seed of a plant native to west Asia. Like all legumes, they have an exceptionally low G.I. value. The reasons include the encapsulation of the starch in a hard seed coat, a higher amylose ratio in the starch and the presence of substances that slow down digestion such as tannins and enzyme inhibitors that aren't destroyed in the cooking process. To cook chickpeas, soak them overnight and then boil them for two to two and one-half hours (or use a pressure cooker). Prepared this way, chickpeas are more fibrous than the canned version and have a lower glycemic index, but both varieties can be used interchangeably.

Chickpeas, Canned and Drained

GLYCEMIC INDEX: 42

■

½ cup boiled chickpeas, drained, contains:

CARBOHYDRATE:	15 g
FAT:	2 g
FIBER:	5 g

Also known as garbanzo beans, chickpeas are the main ingredient in such Middle Eastern specialties as hummus (a cold spreadable puree) and falafel (fried balls or patties). Roasted chickpeas, sprinkled with salt and spices, make a healthy low G.I. snack (see *The Glucose Revolution* [Marlowe & Co., 1999] for an easy, tasty recipe). And although canned chickpeas have a slightly higher glycemic index than the boil-at-home version, they are a quick way for vegetarians (and others) to get a low G.I. source of protein. Canned chickpeas are especially convenient to pop into salads and pita sandwiches for a quick, nutritious, low G.I. lunch.

Kidney Beans, Red, Boiled

GLYCEMIC INDEX: 27

■

½ cup boiled red kidney beans contains:

CARBOHYDRATE:	20 g
FAT:	0 g
FIBER:	7 g

This is the type of bean used in vegetarian and meat chili, as well as in tacos and burritos. This nutrient-packed vegetable protein food has been replaced by the more convenient canned form (see the following entry), with relatively no nutritional loss. Traditionally, dried kidney beans are soaked overnight and can be boiled for two hours without losing their shape or texture. Not only are kidney beans a wonderful addition to Mexican and Tex-Mex cuisines, they make a great side dish for any meal.

Kidney Beans, Red, Canned

GLYCEMIC INDEX: 52

■

½ cup canned red kidney beans contains:

CARBOHYDRATE:	19 g
FAT:	0 g
FIBER:	5 g

Canned kidney beans have a higher glycemic index than home-boiled kidney beans. The high temperatures and/or pressures of the canning process soften the seed casing and induce greater degrees of starch gelatinization of the beans' starch interior, which allows for quicker digestion. Nonetheless, canned kidney beans are a low G.I. food, high in fiber, iron, B vitamins and protein and can make a valuable addition to your diet.

Lentil Soup, Canned

GLYCEMIC INDEX: 44

■

1 cup (8 ounces) contains:

CARBOHYDRATE:	24 g
FAT:	1 g
FIBER:	5 g

Because of the high quality and caloric density of the nutrients in even commercially prepared lentil soup, it qualifies as a meal by itself. Or try pairing it with one of the low G.I. foods on this list (see "Bread" on page 18.) Because both the bread and soup will be slowly digested, the combination will leave you feeling full for hours!

Lentils, Brown

GLYCEMIC INDEX: 30

■

½ cup boiled, dried, brown lentils contains:

CARBOHYDRATE:	16 g
FAT:	0 g
FIBER:	8 g

Legumes are nature's lowest G.I. foods. The reasons include the encapsulation of the starch in a hard seed coat, a higher amylose ratio in the starch and the presence of substances that slow down digestion— such as tannins and enzyme inhibitors—that are not destroyed in the cooking process. They also contain starch that is totally resistant to digestion in the small intestine. Resistant starch behaves like fiber in the large bowel and may reduce the risk of colon cancer.

Lentils are rich in protein, fiber and B vitamins. They are often used as substitutes for meat in vegetarian recipes. The red lentil is one of the oldest known beans. All colors and types of lentils have a similar, low glycemic index, which is increased slightly by canning. They have a fairly bland, earthy flavor and are best prepared with onion, garlic and spices. Whole red lentils fade to yellow with cooking. They cook quickly to mush and are used to make Indian dal (a spiced lentil puree) or curried lentil soup. They are also good for thickening any type of soup or extending meat casseroles.

Lima Beans

GLYCEMIC INDEX: 32

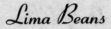

½ cup frozen baby lima beans contains:

CARBOHYDRATE:	17 g
FAT:	0 g
FIBER:	6 g

All legumes, including the lima bean, have a low glycemic index. The lima bean is a large variety of the butter bean. It has a floury texture and slightly sweet flavor. Baby lima beans can be boiled and served as a vegetable beside a serving of meat. Dried and canned lima beans can also be used in soups, stews, casseroles and salads. The reason legumes are nature's lowest G.I. foods is because of the encapsulation of the starch in a hard seed coat, a higher amylose ratio in the starch and the presence of substances that slow down digestion—such as tannins and enzyme inhibitors—that aren't destroyed in the cooking process.

Navy Beans

GLYCEMIC INDEX: 38

■

½ cup boiled dried navy beans contains:

CARBOHYDRATE:	19 g
FAT:	0 g
FIBER:	6 g

Navy beans are used for making baked beans and are an excellent source of fiber, protein, iron, potassium and zinc. If you make your own baked beans, they'll have a lower glycemic index than the canned version. Legumes of all sorts, including navy beans, are renowned for producing flatulence (gas). The components responsible are indigestible sugars called raffinose, stachyose and verbascose. They reach the large bowel intact where they are fermented by the resident microflora. Believe it or not, this is good for colon health, increasing the proportion of good *Bifidobacteria* and reducing the potential pathogens.

Peas, Dried, Split, Yellow or Green

GLYCEMIC INDEX: 22

■

½ cup of boiled, dried split peas contains:

CARBOHYDRATE:	7 g
FAT:	0 g
FIBER:	8 g

All 1,000-plus varieties of peas technically belong to the legume plant family. Dried peas are a storehouse of nutrition and because their calories are slowly digested (low glycemic index) a little of them goes a long way. They take about one hour to cook after soaking and tend to disintegrate if they're over-cooked. Their low glycemic index is due to a combination of factors—higher amylose content, physical entrapment of starch inside the cell wall of the seed, lower levels of starch gelatinization during cooking and higher levels of substances that inhibit enzymes (such as tannins).

Peas, Green

GLYCEMIC INDEX: 48

■

½ cup of fresh green peas, boiled and frozen, contains:

CARBOHYDRATE:	11 g
FAT:	0 g
FIBER:	4 g

Peas are properly classified as legumes. They are high in fiber and also higher in protein than most other vegetables. More amylose, lower degrees of starch gelatinization and protein-starch interactions may contribute to their lower glycemic index. While most of the carbohydrate is starch, they also average 3½ percent sucrose, which gives them a sweet flavor.

Pinto Beans, Canned

GLYCEMIC INDEX: 45

■

½ cup canned pinto beans contains:

CARBOHYDRATE:	18 g
FAT:	1 g
FIBER:	6 g

The canning process slightly raises the glycemic index of pinto beans by permitting greater swelling or gelatinization of the starch molecules, which increases the rate of digestion and absorption. Canned pinto beans still remain, however, a great low G.I. food choice. These versatile beans are used as vegetable side dishes, or added to soups, salads and stews. Their flavor blends particularly well with tomatoes, thyme, oregano, rosemary, mint marjoram, mustard, nutmeg and cardamom.

Pinto Beans, Dried

GLYCEMIC INDEX: 39

■

½ cup dried pinto beans, soaked and boiled, contains:

CARBOHYDRATE:	22 g
FAT:	0 g
FIBER:	7 g

Pinto beans are beige legumes with brown spots ("pinto" is Spanish for "painted") that turn a pinkish hue when you cook them. To prepare these beans, you need to presoak them and cook for one and a half to two hours. Like most members of the legume family, pinto beans are nutritionally and calorically dense. Their high protein, fiber, and resistance to gelatinization all contribute to the pinto bean's low G.I. value.

Soy Beans

GLYCEMIC INDEX: 18

■

½ cup canned soy beans contains:

CARBOHYDRATE:	10 g
FAT:	7 g
FIBER:	5 g

Soy beans contain very good amounts of fiber, iron, zinc and vitamin B and are an excellent source of protein. They are also higher in fat than other legumes, but the majority of this fat is polyunsaturated. They are quite low in carbohydrate. Soy beans also contain phytoestrogens (a type of plant estrogen similar in structure to the female hormone estrogen, but with a much weaker action). Many studies associate soy beans with beneficial effects—improvements in blood cholesterol levels, alleviation of menopausal symptoms, lower risk of breast cancer. (You would need to eat 2 to 3 servings of soy a day to achieve these benefits.) Canned soy beans appear to have a similar glycemic index to their home-cooked counterparts.

You can buy soy beans dried (you'll need to soak and then boil them for about two hours), canned or roasted. You can also enjoy them as soy bean curd (tofu), soy bean flour, tempeh, miso, or textured vegetable protein (TVP), which you can find in veggie burgers. All of these forms of soy beans have little carbohydrate and therefore minimal effect on blood sugar levels. And soy is increasingly popular and available as soy milk (see Vitasoy Soy Milk on page 107).

PASTA

Fettuccine

GLYCEMIC INDEX: 32

■

1 cup of boiled fettucine (2 ounces dry) contains:

CARBOHYDRATE:	57 g
FAT:	1 g
FIBER:	2 g

Fettucine is a ribbon shaped pasta, about ⅛ of an inch wide. It's made from semolina, and dried spinach or eggs may also be added ingredients. It tastes great with cheese-based sauces but it is preferable to use tomato-based accompaniments that have only a fraction of the calories. Pasta's dense consistency makes it resistant to disruption in the small intestine and contributes to the final low glycemic index.

Gnocchi

GLYCEMIC INDEX: 68

■

1 cup cooked gnocchi contains:

CARBOHYDRATE:	71 g
FAT:	3 g
FIBER:	3 g

Gnocchi are small potato dumplings that serve the same function as pasta in Italian cuisine. They may be served with meat, pesto, butter and sage, tomato or rich gorgonzola cream sauces, among others. High calorie sauces, though, warrant smaller portions of gnocchi! There is another type of gnocchi, too, which is made from cornmeal instead of potatoes. This type of gnocchi is generally oven baked rather than boiled.

Macaroni

GLYCEMIC INDEX: 45

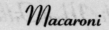

1 cup of boiled macaroni contains:

CARBOHYDRATE:	52 g
FAT:	1 g
FIBER:	3 g

All pastas have a low glycemic index (40 to 50) whatever the shape and no matter how long you cook them. One reason for this is that the making of good pasta starts with wheat semolina (cracked wheat minus the bran) rather than flour. The larger the particle size of the cereal, the slower the rate of gelatinization during cooking, and the slower the rate of digestion in the small intestine. Experiments also show that pasta made with flour tends to have a low glycemic index. The dense texture of all pasta products leads to less disruption during passage through the gastrointestinal tract. Pasta makes a quick and easy meal, especially since there are so many freshly prepared pastas and sauces on the market (it's easy to make your own, too). Stick to the tomato-based sauces rather than the creamy ones laden with fat, and use a modest sprinkling of cheese on top.

Ravioli, Meat-Filled

GLYCEMIC INDEX: 39

■

1 cup of commercial ravioli (meat-filled) contains:

CARBOHYDRATE:	32 g
FAT:	8 g
FIBER:	4 g

You can usually buy ravioli either fresh or vacuum packed, with any number of delicious fillings. A homemade tomato soup topped with floating ravioli and grated Parmesan cheese makes a delicious, low G.I. meal. You can also eat them as a main dish with vegetables and a tomato-based or light butter sauce. Ravioli fillings can also be made from cheese, spinach, tofu, butternut squash, pumpkin, or potatoes.

Spaghetti, White

GLYCEMIC INDEX: 41

■

1 cup of cooked spaghetti contains:

CARBOHYDRATE:	52 g
FAT:	1 g
FIBER:	2 g

Spaghetti is probably the most popular form of pasta. Spaghetti, like all pasta, has a low glycemic index because the starting product is a dough made from high protein semolina (large particles of wheat) and because of its dense food matrix that resists disruption in the small intestine. Both fresh and dried spaghetti have a low glycemic index. Canned spaghetti, which is usually made from flour rather than semolina—and is very well cooked—has a higher glycemic index. Spaghetti's versatility is endless: It blends beautifully with cooked and raw vegetables; any mixture of herbs and spices; meats, poultry, fish and shellfish; and sauces containing oil, margarine, butter or light cream; and even nuts such as walnuts, pine nuts and sunflower seeds.

Spaghetti, Whole Wheat

GLYCEMIC INDEX: 37

■

1 cup of cooked whole wheat spaghetti contains:

CARBOHYDRATE:	48 g
FAT:	1 g
FIBER:	6 g

All the low G.I. virtues of regular enriched spaghetti apply to whole wheat spaghetti and for the same reasons. These two types of pasta can be interchanged in any recipe; you can enjoy this spaghetti with all the same sauces and accompaniments as you would the white. Just keep in mind that you'll be getting more than double the amount of dietary fiber when you eat whole wheat spaghetti instead of white.

Star Pastina

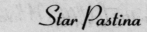

GLYCEMIC INDEX: 38

■

1 cup cooked star-shaped pastina contains:

CARBOHYDRATE:	56 g
FAT:	1 g
FIBER:	2 g

Small pasta or "pastina" comes in many shapes: stars, orzo, acini di pepe, and more. But just like the larger shaped pasta (including spaghetti, macaroni, ziti and elbows) they are all made from durum wheat semolina, which is a low G.I. carbohydrate. Pastinas are used in vegetable, chicken and beef broths to provide some thickeners and added calories to the soup. Children often love the shapes of these smaller pastas.

Tortellini

GLYCEMIC INDEX: 50

■

8 ounces of cheese tortellini with marinara sauce contains:

CARBOHYDRATE:	26 g
FAT:	6 g
FIBER:	1 g

Tortellini is a small, crescent-shaped filled pasta and the range of fillings is unlimited! Some popular fillings include spinach and ricotta, chicken and veal and ham and cheese. Tortellini are usually bought fresh, or vacuum packed, boiled and then served with either a sauce or just grated cheese. The nutrient content will vary depending on the type of filling. Like all pasta, tortellini have a low glycemic index.

RICE

Basmati Rice

GLYCEMIC INDEX: 58

∎

1 cup cooked basmati rice contains:

CARBOHYDRATE:	50 g
FAT:	0 g
FIBER:	0 g

Basmati rice is one of the best known and most used perfumed rices. (Jasmine rice is another popular variety.) Its high content of amylose starch—the kind of starch that breaks down slowly into glucose—is the reason for its low glycemic index. The grains of Basmati rice stay firm and separate when cooked, a characteristic that reflects the compact structure of its starch. You can use this feature to guess the glycemic index values of rices you see on restaurant menus. High amylose rices are preferred in Indian, Thai and Vietnamese cuisines, while rices with less amylose have grains that tend to stick together when cooked, as preferred in Chinese and Italian cuisines. The less amylose there is, the stickier the grains will be and the higher the glycemic index. You can make rice desserts, such as puddings, with Basmati rice.

Brown Rice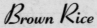

GLYCEMIC INDEX: 55

■

1 cup cooked brown rice contains:

CARBOHYDRATE:	37 g
FAT:	0 g
FIBER:	4 g

Brown rice is the whole rice grain with just the inedible outer shell removed. Brown rice is the most nutritious form of rice, because it contains several B vitamins and minerals, dietary fiber and protein. Its compact structure and fibrous nature make it an excellent low G.I. food choice. Since it's much more chewy than regular white rice, eating brown rice in your favorite dishes may take some getting used to. But once you've made the switch you'll find that it's a delicious and hearty side dish or main dish ingredient.

Long Grain White Rice

GLYCEMIC INDEX: 56

■

1 cup cooked long grain white rice contains:

CARBOHYDRATE:	42 g
FAT:	0 g
FIBER:	1 g

Long grain rice is light and delicate. One bonus for cooks is that the grains also remain separate when they're cooked. No more clumps! Like the other low G.I. rices, the compact structure and high amylose starch content contribute to long grain rice's slow digestion rate. Delicious as a side dish, many people also add long grain white rice to casseroles and use them to make cold rice salads, as well.

Uncle Ben's Converted ™ *Rice*

GLYCEMIC INDEX: 44

■

1 cup of Uncle Ben's Converted Rice contains:

CARBOHYDRATE:	38 g
FAT:	0 g
FIBER:	1 g

Parboiled or converted long grain white rice is soaked, then steamed, before being milled. This process transfers the B vitamins and minerals that are contained in the germ and outer layers to the interior of the grain. Converted or parboiled rice is second only to brown rice in its nutritional quality. In addition, its high amylose starch content gives it its low glycemic index. You can use parboiled rice in any of the same ways (and in the same dishes) as you would other types of rice.

SNACKS, DESSERTS AND BEVERAGES

Custard

GLYCEMIC INDEX: 43

■

½ cup of custard contains:

CARBOHYDRATE:	24 g
FAT:	4 g
FIBER:	0 g

Custard is prepared from commercial wheat starch with egg, milk and sugar added. Its low glycemic index may be explained by its fat content (which slows down stomach emptying) and its sugars, sucrose and lactose, which have only half the glycemic effect of pure wheat starch. Custard makes a creamy, sweet low G.I. dessert. Sprinkle a little nutmeg on top for an old-fashioned look and taste.

Granola Bar, Quaker Chewy ™

GLYCEMIC INDEX: 61

■

1 1-ounce Granola Bar contains:

CARBOHYDRATE:	23 g
FAT:	2 g
FIBER:	1 g

This snack bar is made from whole grain rolled oats and whole grain rolled wheat. The 18 grams of sugar in each bar come from the natural sugars in the added fruits (such as raisins and apples) and from sucrose. "Rolled" grains have been hulled and rolled to produce flat flakes, helping to make this a compact snack bar. A nutritious low G.I. snack, Quaker Chewy Granola Bars can double as a quick on-the-run breakfast when you combine it with a container of light yogurt or a glass of skim milk and a piece of fruit.

Oatmeal Cookie

GLYCEMIC INDEX: 55

■

1 cookie (⅔ ounce) contains:

CARBOHYDRATE:	12 g
FAT:	3 g
FIBER:	less than 1 g

The use of rolled oats, along with some sugar and added fat is probably why oatmeal cookies have such a low glycemic index. Nutritionists explain that there is, in fact, a place for cookies in a balanced meal plan as long as the portion you choose is a small one. Oatmeal cookies would make an excellent low G.I. choice for a sweet and tasty dessert.

Popcorn, Light Microwave

GLYCEMIC INDEX: 55

∎

2 cups popped light microwave popcorn contains:

CARBOHYDRATE:	12 g
FAT:	3 g
FIBER:	2 g

Popcorn is made from a special type of corn in which high heat causes the kernels to expand with steam and burst open, which then exposes the starchy center of the grain. It has a surprisingly low glycemic index considering that popping gives other products a very high glycemic index. The reason for its low G.I. value could be because the corn has a low moisture content to start with, which may inhibit starch gelatinization. Popcorn contains a reasonable amount of fiber and can be low in fat (depending on preparation). Read labels carefully to make sure you're choosing a low fat product. (See "Are You Really Choosing Low Fat" on page 15 for some label-reading guidelines.)

Power Bar ™ Performance Chocolate Bar

GLYCEMIC INDEX: 58

∎

1 2.8-ounce bar contains:

CARBOHYDRATE:	45 g
FAT:	2 g
FIBER:	3 g

With over 200 calories contained it its 2 to 3 ounces, the Power Bar is an energy-dense bar formulated with an athlete's energy needs in mind. The carbohydrate sources have low to intermediate glycemic index values. The fiber and the fat also contribute to a more prolonged digestion of these nutrients, which means that Power Bars give athletes a longer lasting energy source from which to draw during workouts or athletic events.

Pudding, Cooked, Sugar Free

GLYCEMIC INDEX: 43

∎

½ cup cooked pudding contains:

CARBOHYDRATE:	24 g
FAT:	4 g
FIBER:	0 g

When cooked with whole milk, sugar free pudding in any flavor is a sweet tasting, nutritious, low G.I. dessert that provides 150 mg of calcium. Because the primary carbohydrate source (cornstarch) has not been modified to reduce the cooking time, the chemical breakdown into glucose is slower, which is why cooked puddings have lower G.I. values than instant varieties. If you're looking for a sweet, low G.I. dessert idea, sugar free puddings might be the answer.

Social Tea Biscuits ™ (Nabisco)

GLYCEMIC INDEX: 55

•

4 Social Tea biscuits contain:

CARBOHYDRATE:	13 g
FAT:	3 g
FIBER:	1 g

Social Tea biscuits aren't biscuits as we know them; in fact, they're thin, sweet little cookies. What makes this a low G.I. snack? Cookie doughs have a low water-to-flour ratio and a high sugar content, which results in lower levels of starch gelatinization than in most bread doughs. All things considered, cookies, whether high or low in sugar, are packed with calories and taste great, so it's easy to overeat them. Eat these in moderation.

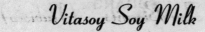

Vitasoy Soy Milk

GLYCEMIC INDEX: 31

■

1 cup (8 ounces) of creamy original Vitasoy soy milk contains:

CARBOHYDRATE:	14 g
FAT:	7 g
FIBER:	1 g

Soy milk is a completely dairy- and lactose-free milk. Whole soybeans—which are often organically grown—are mixed with filtered water and flavorings to produce a milk-like product. Once enjoyed only by vegetarians, soy milk is becoming increasingly popular, possibly because it is a rich source of isoflavones, nutrients which are known to have health benefits. (See the "Soy Beans" entry on page 87 for more information about these benefits.)

SUGARS

Fructose

GLYCEMIC INDEX: 23

■

3 packets contains:

CARBOHYDRATE:	10 g
FAT:	0 g
FIBER:	0 g

Fructose (or fruit sugar) is a form of sugar that occurs naturally in all fruits and honey. Apples are a particularly rich source of free fructose. Fructose is also found as one half of the sucrose (refined sugar) molecule.

Fructose is slowly absorbed into the bloodstream and only gradually converted to glucose in the liver. Its presence in the liver brings about a prompt reduction in the body's normal glucose-producing mechanisms (something that glucose doesn't do). All in all, fructose has only 20 percent of the effect of pure glucose on blood sugar and insulin levels. Some studies show that very large amounts of fructose have undesirable effects on blood fats, but in normal everyday amounts that we find in most foods, there is no cause for concern.

Honey

GLYCEMIC INDEX: 58

■

1 tablespoon contains:

CARBOHYDRATE:	16 g
FAT:	0 g
FIBER:	0 g

Honey is a concentrated source of carbohydrate and is basically a mixture of glucose and fructose. Honey's glycemic index appears to be similar to that of refined sugar (about 60), unless it is glucose enriched (which increases its glycemic index). Honey was a major source of sweetness at the beginning of the nineteenth century—long before refined sugar became available. In fact, historical research suggests that in some parts of the world people ate quantities of honey similar to the amount of refined sugar we now eat. There are negligible quantities of other nutrients in honey.

Lactose

GLYCEMIC INDEX: 46

■

⁷/₁₀ of an ounce of pure lactose contains:

CARBOHYDRATE:	10 g
FAT:	0 g
FIBER:	0 g

Lactose is a disaccharide ("double sugar") that needs to be digested into its component sugars before the body can absorb it. The two sugars, glucose and galactose, compete with each other for absorption. Once absorbed, galactose is mainly metabolized in the liver producing little effect on plasma glucose levels. So ingesting about 1½ ounces of lactose is equivalent to consuming less than 1 ounce of glucose, and the effect on blood glucose levels is proportionately lower.

For many years people with diabetes were advised to avoid all sugars, which for some, led to the restriction of milk, because of its lactose content. This is no longer considered necessary. Furthermore, milk is an important source of calcium from birth through old age. Some people are lactose intolerant because the enzyme lactase is no longer active in their small intestine, but that should not stop them from enjoying lactose-reduced or lactose-free milk throughout the day. Lactose intolerant people can usually tolerate yogurt because the microorganisms in the yogurt are active in digesting lactose during passage through the small intestine. Cheese is a good source of calcium, too, that is virtually free of lactose.

VEGETABLES

Corn, Canned and Drained

GLYCEMIC INDEX: 55

■

½ cup canned corn, drained, contains:

CARBOHYDRATE:	15 g
FAT:	1 g
FIBER:	2 g

Sweet corn contains folic acid, potassium, the antioxidant vitamins A and C and dietary fiber. In addition to using canned corn in soups, mixed vegetables, stews, relishes and salads, manufacturers use fresh corn to make tortillas, hominy grits, polenta, corn bread, cornflakes and corn oil. Topped with just a hint of butter, corn makes an excellent side dish.

New Potatoes, Canned

GLYCEMIC INDEX: 61

∎

5 small cocktail-size canned new potatoes contain:

CARBOHYDRATE:	23 g
FAT:	0 g
FIBER:	2 g

Canned new potatoes are the smallest potatoes available in the supermarket. These potatoes are already boiled and ready to use in stews or soups or as a tasty side dish. It's a good idea to keep a few cans of these new potatoes on hand in the pantry for those nights when you're not sure what side dish to serve for dinner. All you have to do is open the can and you have a convenient, easy-to-prepare low G.I. dish all ready to go.

New Potatoes, Fresh

GLYCEMIC INDEX: 62

■

5 small cocktail-size boiled new potatoes contain:

CARBOHYDRATE:	23 g
FAT:	0 g
FIBER:	4 g

Most potatoes have a high glycemic index but small new potatoes appear to be the exception. In fact, we found that the smaller the potato, the lower the glycemic index. They are also known as cocktail potatoes. They are good to steam, boil or include in a potato salad. The relatively low glycemic index (compared to the mature potato) results from the lack of branching in the amylopectin starch. As the potato matures and grows bigger, the amylopectin becomes increasingly branched, making it easier to gelatinize during cooking. The branching of the molecule increases the openness of the granules and inhibits bonding between chains of starch. Water is absorbed more easily and the starch granule swells (gelatinizes) at lower temperatures. Gelatinized starch granules are easier to digest.

POTATOES—WHICH TO CHOOSE

Boiled, mashed, baked or in chips—everyone loves potatoes in some form or another. Unfortunately, recent tests have confirmed that the humble spud has a high G.I. value (greater than 78). The only potatoes found to bear anything close to a low glycemic index were the tiny new variety. The lower glycemic index of new potatoes may be due to differences in the structure of the starch. As potatoes age, the degree of branching of their amylopectin starch increases significantly, becoming more readily gelatinized and digested, which produces a higher glycemic index. New potatoes are also smaller than mature potatoes and scientists have found a correlation between the size of the potato and its G.I. value—the smaller the potato, the lower the glycemic index.

So, we suggest eating small, new potatoes and putting the low G.I. focus on the other meals in your day. Vary your diet with other sources of carbohydrate—rice, pasta, legumes. And remember, potatoes are fat free, nutritious and very satisfying. Not everything has to have a low glycemic index—enjoy them!

Sweet Potato

GLYCEMIC INDEX: 54

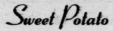

½ cup of mashed sweet potato contains:

CARBOHYDRATE:	20 g
FAT:	0 g
FIBER:	3 g

The orange colored sweet potato is an excellent source of beta-carotene, the plant precursor of vitamin A. Sweet potato is also a good source of vitamin C and fiber. The sweet flavor comes from naturally present sucrose (3 percent), which increases during storage in warm climates to as much as 6 percent. The low glycemic index is associated with increased amounts of amylose.

Sweet potatoes belong to a different plant family than the regular white potatoes and have a much lower glycemic index. Prepare and cook them as you would ordinary potatoes—steam, boil, mash, bake or fry them. They're also tasty additions to casseroles, curries and soups.

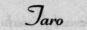

Taro

GLYCEMIC INDEX: 54

■

½ cup of cooked taro contains:

CARBOHYDRATE:	23 g
FAT:	0 g
FIBER:	3 g

Taro is the large tuber of a tropical climbing plant. It has a dry textured flesh and its flavor is not unlike sweet potato. It is slowly digested because of increased amounts of amylose starch. The tubers contain calcium oxalate, which tastes bitter if eaten raw. Be sure to peel off a thick portion of the taro's skin before cooking, and protect your own skin with rubber gloves. You can then cook it as you would a potato—steamed, boiled or baked.

Tomato Soup

GLYCEMIC INDEX: 38

■

1 cup of canned tomato soup, prepared, contains:

CARBOHYDRATE:	33 g
FAT:	4 g
FIBER:	1 g

Canned tomato soups tend to contain large amounts of sodium, so look for salt-reduced varieties when purchasing your next can. Besides making an easy meal with some low G.I. toast, tomato soup can be used undiluted in many casserole recipes. The low glycemic index is related to its acidity and the bulk of its carbohydrate being sucrose.

Yam

GLYCEMIC INDEX: 51

∎

3 ounces of boiled/baked yam contains:

CARBOHYDRATE:	25 g
FAT:	0 g
FIBER:	3 g

The edible roots of climbing plants, yams are a good source of vitamin C and potassium. They are similar to sweet potato and can be prepared in similar ways—boiled, baked or deep fried. In fact, you can eat yams in place of sweet or white potatoes in most recipes. The low glycemic index is related to a higher proportion of amylose in the starch fraction.

GLYCEMIC INDEX TESTING

If you are a food manufacturer, you may be interested in having the glycemic index of some of your products tested on a fee-for-service basis. For more information, contact either:

Glycaemic Index Testing Inc.
135 Mavety Street
Toronto, Ontario
Canada M6P 2L8
E-mail: thomas.wolever@utoronto.ca

or

Sydney University Glycaemic Index Research Service (SUGIRS)
Department of Biochemistry
University of Sydney
NSW 2006 Australia
Fax: (61) (2) 9351-6022
E-mail: j.brandmiller@staff.usyd.edu.au

FOR MORE INFORMATION

REGISTERED DIETITIANS

Registered Dietitians (R.D.s) are nutrition experts who provide nutritional assessment and guidance. Check for the initials "R.D." after the name to identify qualified dietitians who provide the highest standard of care to their clients. The glycemic index is part of their training so all dietitians should be able to help in applying the principles in this guide, but some dietitians do specialize in certain areas. If you want more detailed advice on the glycemic index just ask the dietitian whether this is a specialty when you make your appointment.

Dietitians work in hospitals and often run their own private practices, as well. For a list of dietitians in your area, contact the American Dietetic Association (ADA) Consumer Nutrition Hotline (1-800-366-1655) or visit ADA's home page at the address below. You can also check the Yellow Pages under "Dietitians."

The American Dietetic Association
216 West Jackson Boulevard
Chicago, IL 60606
Phone: 1-800-877-1600
Fax: 1-312-899-1979
Web site: http://www.eatright.org/

NATURAL OVENS ORDERING INFORMATION

Natural Ovens of Manitowoc
4300 County Trunk CR
P.O. Box 730
Manitowoc, WI 54221-0730
Telephone: 1-800-772-0730
Fax: 920-758-2594
http://www.naturalovens.com/

ACKNOWLEDGMENTS

We would like to acknowledge the extraordinary efforts of Johanna Burani and Linda Rao, who adapted this book—and the other books in *The Glucose Revolution Pocket Guide* series—for North American readers. Together they have worked to ensure that every piece of information is accurate and appropriate for readers in the U.S. and Canada.

ABOUT THE AUTHORS

Kaye Foster-Powell, B.Sc., M. Nutr. & Diet., is an accredited dietitian-nutritionist in both public and private practice in New South Wales, Australia. A graduate of the University of Sydney (B.Sc., 1987; Masters of Nutrition and Dietetics, 1994), she has extensive experience in diabetes management and has researched practical applications of the glycemic index over the last five years. A co-author of *The Glucose Revolution* and all the titles in *The Glucose Revolution Pocket Guide* Series, she lives in Sydney, Australia.

Jennie Brand-Miller, Ph.D., Associate Professor of Human Nutrition in the Human Nutrition Unit, Department of Biochemistry, University of Sydney, Australia, is widely recognized as one of the world's leading authorities on the glycemic index. She received her B.Sc. (1975) and Ph.D. (1979) degrees from the Department of Food Science and Technology at the University of New South Wales, Australia. She is the editor of the *Proceedings of the Nutrition Society of Australia* and a member of the Scientific Consultative Committee of the Australian Nutrition Foundation. She has written more than 200 research papers, including 60 on the glycemic index of foods. A co-author of *The Glucose*

Revolution and all the titles in *The Glucose Revolution Pocket Guide* Series, she lives in Sydney, Australia.

Thomas M.S. Wolever, M.D., Ph.D., another of the world's leading researchers of the glycemic index, is Professor in the Department of Nutritional Sciences, University of Toronto, and a member of the Division of Endocrinology and Metabolism, St. Michael's Hospital, Toronto. He is a graduate of Oxford University (B.A., M.A., M.B., B.Ch., M.Sc., and D.M.). He received his Ph.D. at the University of Toronto. His research since 1980 has focused on the glycemic index of foods and the prevention of type 2 diabetes. A co-author of *The Glucose Revolution* and all the titles in *The Glucose Revolution Pocket Guide* Series, he lives in Toronto, Canada.

Johanna Burani, M.S., R.D., C.D.E., is a registered dietitian and certified diabetes educator with more than 10 years experience in nutritional counseling. She specializes in designing individual meal plans based on low glycemic-index food choices. The adapter of *The Glucose Revolution* and co-adapter, with Linda Rao, of all the titles in *The Glucose Revolution Pocket Guide* Series, she is the author of seven books and professional manuals, and lives in Mendham, New Jersey.

Linda Rao, M.Ed., a freelance writer and editor, has been writing and researching health topics for the past 11 years. Her work has appeared in several national publications, including *Prevention* and *USA*

Today. She serves as a contributing editor for *Prevention* Magazine and is the co-adapter, with Johanna Burani, of all the titles in *The Glucose Revolution Pocket Guide* Series. She lives in Allentown, Pennsylvania.

INDEX

25.	Cherries	57
26.	Chickpeas, boiled	75
27.	Chickpeas, canned and drained	42
28.	Cookie, oatmeal	102
29.	Corn, canned and drained	111
30.	Couscous	42
31.	Cream of Wheat, Old Fashioned	31
32.	Custard	100
33.	Fettucine	88
34.	Fructose	108
35.	Fruit cocktail	58
36.	Gnocchi	89
37.	Granola bar, Quaker Chewy™	101
38.	Grapefruit	59
39.	Grapefruit juice	60
40.	Grapes, green	61
41.	Honey	109
42.	Ice cream, low fat	45
43.	Kidney beans, red, boiled	77
44.	Kidney beans, red, canned	78
45.	Kiwi	62
46.	Lactose	110
47.	Lentil soup, canned	79
48.	Lentils, brown	80
49.	Lima beans	81
50.	Macaroni	90
51.	Mango	63
52.	Milk, chocolate, 1% milk fat	46
53.	Milk, skim	47
54.	Milk, whole	48
55.	Muesli, natural	32
56.	Muesli, toasted	33
57.	Multi-Bran Chex™, General Mills	34
58.	Navy beans	82
59.	Oat bran, raw	43

60. Oat bran breakfast cereal, Quaker Oats™	35
61. Oatmeal, Old Fashioned	36
62. Orange, navel	64
63. Papaya	65
64. Peach, canned, natural juice	66
65. Peach, fresh	67
66. Pear, canned, natural juice	68
67. Pear, fresh	69
68. Peas, dried split, yellow or green	83
69. Peas, green, frozen	84
70. Pinto beans, dried	86
71. Pinto beans, canned	85
72. Plum	70
73. Popcorn, light microwave	103
74. Potatoes, new, fresh	113
75. Potatoes, new, canned	112
76. Power Bar™, Performance Chocolate Bar	104
77. Pudding, cooked, sugar free	105
78. Pumpernickel bread	24
79. Ravioli, meat-filled, cooked	91
80. Rice bran	44
81. Rice, Basmati	96
82. Rice, brown	97
83. Rice, Converted™, Uncle Ben's	99
84. Rice, long grain white	98
85. Shredded Wheat, Post™	37
86. Social Tea biscuits™, Nabisco	106
87. Soy beans	87
88. Spaghetti, white	92
89. Spaghetti, whole wheat	93
90. Special K™, Kellogg's, breakfast cereal	38
91. Star Pastina	94
92. Sweet potato	115
93. Taro	116
94. Tomato soup, canned	117

95. Tortellini, cheese   95
96. Vitasoy soy milk   107
97. Yam, boiled, baked   118
98. Yogurt, nonfat, fruit flavored, artificial sweetener   49
99. Yogurt, nonfat, fruit flavored, with sugar   50
100. Yogurt, nonfat, plain   51

You can find a complete listing of all tested foods and their G.I.   values in *The Glucose Revolution* (Marlowe & Co., 1999).

The Glucose Revolution begins here . . .

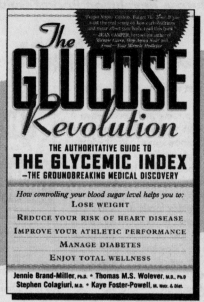

THE GLUCOSE REVOLUTION
THE AUTHORITATIVE GUIDE TO THE GLYCEMIC INDEX—
THE GROUNDBREAKING MEDICAL DISCOVERY

NATIONAL BESTSELLER!

"Forget *Sugar Busters*. Forget *The Zone*. If you want the real scoop on how carbohydrates and sugar affect your body, read this book by the world's leading researchers on the subject. It's the authoritative, last word on choosing foods to control your blood sugar."

—JEAN CARPER, best-selling author of *Miracle Brain, Miracle Cures, Stop Aging Now!* and *Food—Your Miracle Medicine*

ISBN 1-56924-660-2 • $14.95

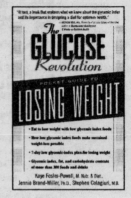
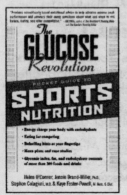

The Glucose Revolution Pocket Guide to
DIABETES

Help control your diabetes with low glycemic index foods

Based on the most up-to-date information about carbohydrates, this basic guide to the glycemic index and diabetes allows people with type 1 and type 2 diabetes to make more informed choices about their diets. Topics covered include why many traditionally "taboo" foods don't cause the unfavorable effects on blood sugar levels they were believed to have, and why diets based on low G.I. foods improve blood sugar control. Also covered are how to include more of the right kinds of carbohydrates in your diet, the

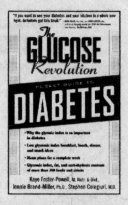

optimum diet for people with diabetes, practical hints for meal preparation and tips to help make the glycemic index work throughout the day, a week of low G.I. menus, G.I. success stories, and more.

ISBN 1-56924-675-0 • $4.95

The Glucose Revolution Pocket Guide to
SUGAR AND ENERGY

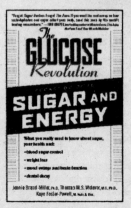

Sugar's off the black list—find out why

Based on the most up-to-date information about carbohydrates, this basic guide to the glycemic index dispels many common myths about sugar and why it's high time to get rid of the guilt. With evidence showing that restricting refined sugar in your diet may do more harm than good, the authors show you how to intelligently give in to your sugar cravings and regulate your sugar intake to control your blood sugar level and lose weight, with the glycemic index for nearly 150 foods.

ISBN 1-56924-641-6 • $4.95

Forthcoming June 2000

The Glucose Revolution Pocket Guide to
YOUR HEART

Healthy eating you can feel in your heart

The latest medical research clearly con-
firms that slowly digested low G.I. carbohydrates like pasta, grainy breads,
cereals based on wheat bran and oats,
and many popular Mediterranean-style
foods play an important part in treating
and preventing heart disease—in addition to controlling blood sugar and aid-
ing weight loss. With 21 pages of
charts, this handy pocket guide shows
you how to choose the right amount of
the right carbohydrates for reducing the
risk of heart attack and for lifelong health
and wellbeing.

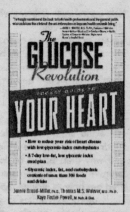

ISBN 1-56924-640-8 • $4.95

Forthcoming June 2000